This Page is intentionally left blank

30

RECIPES AND FORMULA

TO STOP

HIGH BLOOD PRESSURE

BY

ADEDDOYIN S.T (B.PHARM)

TABLE OF CONTENT

This Page is intentionally left blank

INTRODUCTION

Thank you for purchasing this book. My main goal of writing e-books is to proffer solution to various health challenges (which are otherwise difficult to treat) of individuals.

This book is all about using prescribed diet to reduce your high blood pressure in order to increase your quality of life.

My name is Pharm. Samuel Adedoyin. I want to encourage you to read this book from the beginning to the end and apply all the information in it. I promise you will not regret it.

In this book, I am going to show you the powerful benefits of controlled diet in the prevention and management of hypertension. This controlled diet is known as DASH Diet.

WHAT IS DASH DIET?

DASH is an acronym for Dietary Approach to Stop Hypertension.

DASH diet is a dietary pattern (healthy way) to control and prevent hypertension and it is promoted by National Heart, Lung and Blood Institute, United States.

It is a way in which hypertension can be prevented. It encourages you to take a diet rich in potassium, calcium and magnesium and reduce intake of sodium in your diet.

Also, DASH diet is rich in vegetables, whole grains, fruits, fish, meat, poultry, nuts, beans and low fat dairy products and the good news is that it can be adapted to your favorite foods, taste and lifestyle.

It has been scientifically established that blood pressure can be lowered by following the DASH eating plan, and by reducing salt intake, also called sodium.

DASH diet also prevents osteoporosis (a condition in which the bone becomes weak and break easily), cancer, heart disease, stroke and diabetes, as it has a high amount of antioxidant rich food.

WHAT YOU NEED TO KNOW ABOUT HYPERTENSION

The number one risk factor for death world is high blood pressure.

Hypertension, or high blood pressure refers to the pressure of blood against your arterial (blood vessels) walls. Over time, high blood pressure can cause blood vessel damage that leads to heart disease, kidney disease, stroke, and other problems.

Hypertension is sometimes called the silent killer because it produces no symptoms and can go unnoticed and untreated for years.

Whenever you check your blood pressure in your clinic or any hospital, and the reading is 140/90mmHg in more than 3 consecutive occasions, it simply means that you have hypertension and must be controlled to the normal blood pressure.

The normal blood pressure is below 120/80 mmHg. The upper reading is called the systolic, while the lower reading is called the diastolic blood pressures respectively.

If your blood pressure is above 120/80mmHg, you do not necessarily have hypertension but you will need to lower it, to maintain a good health.

Of course, hypertension can be managed with anti-hypertensive drugs. In fact, as a pharmacist, I know all the drugs used for the management of hypertension. The problem about these drugs is that they are chemicals and as such, they all have undesirable side effects. This side effects are cumulative. In order words, the higher the doses of your drugs, the greater the side effects. So if your blood pressure (BP) is too

high, you will need more drugs at higher doses to reduce the BP, and definitely, you will experience greater side effects.

The Dash method involves the use of only food components which are natural products without any undesirable side effects.

Please note that I am not saying you shouldn't take anti-hypertensive drugs for established hypertension. In fact, they are very important and you should be placed on them by a licensed medical doctor.

This is what I am saying in essence. By adopting this DASH method, you will be able to prevent hypertension, and if you already have hypertension, your BP will reduce significantly and you will be able to reduce the number and dosage of drugs you need to maintain normal BP and a good health.

Sometimes one may have hypertension that is difficult to control with drugs alone. Adopting DASH method, with physical exercise and reducing salt intake will go a long way to control the BP.

Having said that, I am sure you now have an idea of how this diet could improve your overall quality of life and give you a good health and a happy life.

This Page is intentionally left blank

THE DASH EATING PLAN

The table below gives the daily serving and quantity needed for all classes of food to qualify as a DASH Diet

CLASS OF FOOD	DASH DAILY SERVING	DASH SERVING SIZE
FRUITS	4–5	1 medium piece of fruit or 1/4 cup dried fruit or ½ cup fresh, frozen or canned fruit
VEGETABLES	4–5	250 ml (1 cup) of raw leafy vegetables or ½ cup cooked vegetables or 170 ml of juice.
GRAINS (WHHOLE GRAINS)	6–8	1 sliced bread or 1 cup of ready to eat cereal or ½ cup of cooked rice, pasta or cereal
FAT-FREE OR LOWFAT MILK AND DAIRY	2–3	1 cup of milk or 1 cup of yoghurt
PROTEINS (LEAN MEAT, FISH AND POULTRY)	2 or less	84 grams cooked lean meats, skinless poultry , or fish
NUTS (SEEDS AND LEGUMES)	4–5 per week	1/3 cup nuts or ½ cups cooked dried beans or pea
OILS (PALM AND VEGETABLE)	2–3	5 ml of soft margarine or 5 ml of vegetable oil or 15 ml of of low-fat mayonnaise or 30 ml of light salad dressing

It is not enough to know the classes of food which the DASH Diet comprises. The right quantity makes it work for the purpose intended.

SO PLEASE, AND PLEASE, DO NOT UNDERESTIMATE THE DAILY SERVING AND SERVING SIZES.

This means you must calculate/ measure the quantity required for your chosen recipes

This is a 250 ml cup. You can get this in the market at a cheap price for measuring the quantity of each recipe needed according to the table above.

1 cup = 250 ml; ½ cup = 125 ml (i.e the line between 100 and 150 ml), etc. This calculation is very simple.

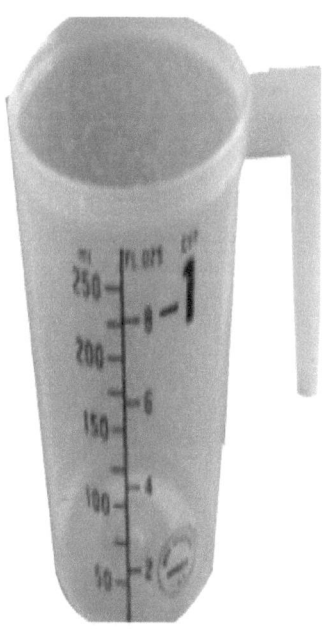

We shall now discuss these classes one by one; and how to go about preparing the right quantities and adapting to your favorite foods.

FRUITS

All fruits are rich in fibre, potassium, magnesium and low in fat except avocado and coconut. To be in line with the DASH guideline, you must take 4-5 servings of this per day. One serving can be 1 medium piece of fruit or ¼ cup dried fruit or ½ cup fresh, frozen or canned fruit. You can choose any of the 3 recipes as desired.

This implies that in order to take four servings a day, you will have to take either 1 medium piece of fruit four times daily or ¼ cup (63 ml) dried fruit four times a day or ½ cup (125 ml) fresh, frozen or canned fruit, four times a day.

The above explanation applies to all other food classes on the table above. Just follow the table. Some best examples of the fruits that can be taken for this purpose include bananas, apples, oranges, tangerine, strawberry, watermelon, African cherry, , blueberries, date fruit,

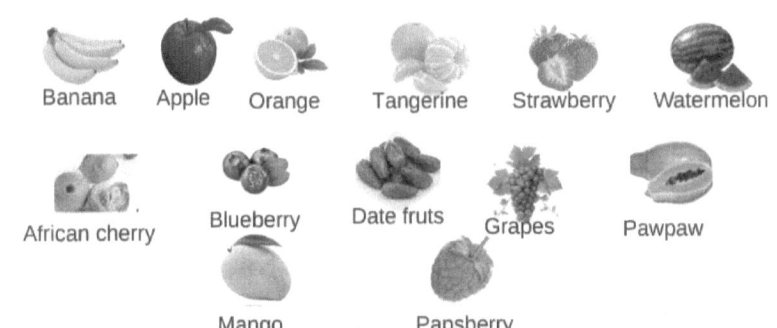

Banana   Apple   Orange   Tangerine   Strawberry   Watermelon

African cherry   Blueberry   Date fruts   Grapes   Pawpaw

Mango   .   Papsberry

grapes, pawpaw, mangoes and raspberry.

VEGETABLES

Raw tomatoes and green leafy vegetables contains diverse vitamins and minerals. They also help in increasing production of a chemical agent called nitric oxide in the body (which increases the size of the blood vessels and

> To be in line with the DASH guideline, you must take 4-5 servings per day.
>
> One serving can either be 250 ml (1 cup) of raw leafy vegetables or ½ cup cooked vegetables or 170 ml of juice.

thus, allow free flow of blood, thereby reduces blood pressure).

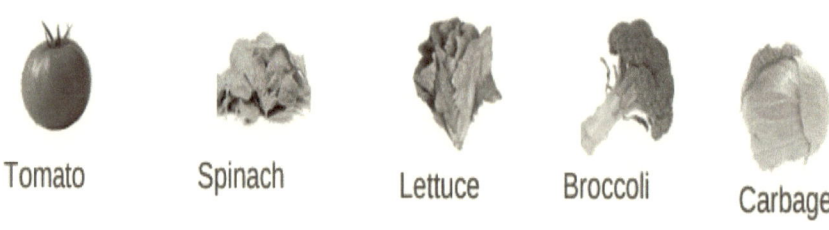

Tomato   Spinach   Lettuce   Broccoli   Carbage

Examples of green leafy vegetables are spinach, lettuce, broccoli cabbage. The list is endless.

GRAINS (WHOLE GRAINS)

Here focus should be on whole wheat pasta, brown rice, barley, oats and whole grain bread.

White rice should be replaced with brown rice.

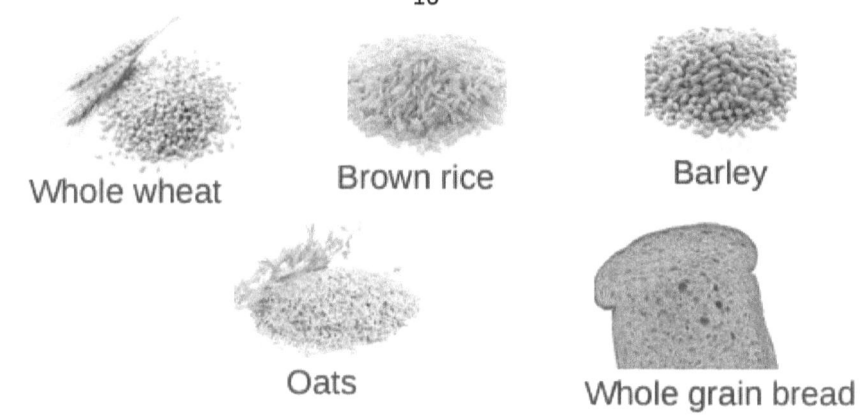

Whole wheat

Brown rice

Barley

Oats

Whole grain bread

Please avoid using cheese, cream or butter.

FAT-FREE OR LOWFAT MILK AND DAIRY

To be in line with the DASH guideline, you must take 6-8 servings of this per day.

One serving can be 1 sliced bread or 1 cup of ready to eat cereal or ½ cup of cooked rice, pasta or cereal

Dairy products like milk, yoghurt and cheese are rich in calcium, protein and vitamin D.

PROTEINS (LEAN MEAT, FISH AND POULTRY)

Meat is a rich source of iron, proteins, B vitamins and zinc.Fishes such as salmon, herring and tuna are rich in omega-3- fatty acids

(Omega-3 fatty acids are essential nutrients that are

To be in line with the DASH guideline, you have to take 2-3 servings of this per day.

One serving can be 1 cup of milk or 1 cup of yoghurt. Fat-free cheeses are high in sodium, so be careful to take just little or avoid totally.

important in preventing and managing heart disease. Findings show omega-3 fatty acids helps to Lower blood pressure.)

Findings have shown that the skin of poultry and meat contain bad cholesterol (known as low density lipoprotein cholesterol) which when eaten, are deposited in the wall of the blood vessels. This gradually, degrade the blood vessels , causing increase in blood pressure and may lead to stroke.

Instead of frying in fat, trim away skin and fat from poultry and meat, and bake, broil, roast or grill meat and poultry.

Soya beans like tofu have all aminoacids (which are needed for vital processes like the building of proteins and synthesis of hormones and neurotransmitters) and can be an alternative source to meat.

To be in line with the DASH guideline, you must take 2 servings or less per day.

One serving can be 84 grams cooked lean meats, skinless poultry, or fish.

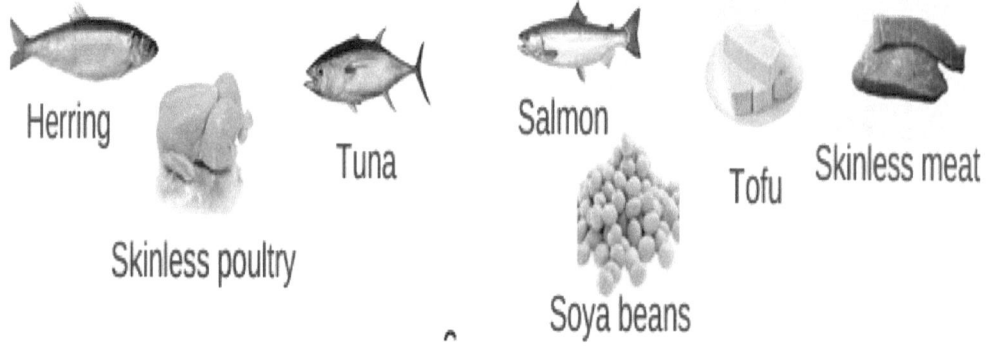

Herring

Skinless poultry

Tuna

Salmon

Soya beans

Tofu

Skinless meat

NUTS (SEEDS AND LEGUMES)

Seeds like almonds, kidney beans, peas, lentils, sunflower seeds and flax seeds are a good source of magnesium, protein and potassium.

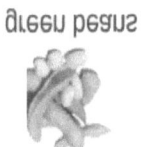 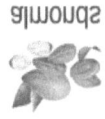 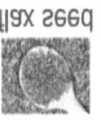 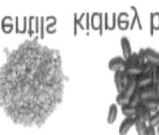

green beans   almonds   flax seeds   lentils   kidney beans

These seeds have medicinal chemicals and dietary fibres that reduce high blood pressure and protect against cardiovascular diseases and cancers.

OILS (PALM AND VEGETABLE OILS)

DASH Diet limits the daily saturated fat intake to less than 6 % of total calories by limiting the use of whole milk, cream, eggs, butter, cheese, coconut and plam oils.

Please avoid foods like fried items, and crackers which have a lot of transfat in them.

To be in line with the DASH guideline, you must take 2 servings or less per day.

One serving can be 5 ml of soft margarine or 5 ml of vegetable oil or 15 ml of of low-fat mayonnaise or 30 ml of light salad dressing.

From the table above you can prepare a table of balanced DASH diet as you desire.

To be in line with the DASH guideline, you must take 6-8 servings per week.

One serving can be 1/3 cup nuts or ½ cups cooked dried beans or peas.

Now, using the formula in the table above, I have prepared a sample of what I called the balanced DASH DIET for 7

DAYS	BREAKFAST	LUNCH	SUPER
1	2 cups of cooked brown rice with 5 ml of palm oil +1½ cup cooked vegetables + 1 cup of fruit juice	1 cup of yoghurt	2 cups cooked vegetables with 15 ml of palm oil +1/2 piece herring fish +1 apple+ 2 bananas
2	7 slices of bread + 1 cup of milk	1 cups of cooked brown rice with 5 ml of palm oil + ½ cup cooked vegetables + a piece of skinless meat + 1 cup of fruit juice	½ cup of cooked dried beans with 5ml of palm oil +2 cups of yoghurt
3	3 slices of bread + 1 cup of milk	½ cup of cooked dried beans with 5ml of palm oil +1 orange + 2 bananas	2 cups cooked vegetables with 10 ml of palm oil + ½ piece fish + 1 cup of cooked brown rice + 1 cup of yoghurt
4	½ cup of cooked dried beans with 5 ml of palm oil +1 cup of fruit juice	2 cups of cooked brown rice +1½ cup cooked vegetables with 5 ml of palm oil + 2 cups of yoghurt	1 cups of cooked brown rice + ½ cup cooked vegetables with 10 ml of palm oil + a piece of skinless poultry + 1 cup of fruit juice
5	4 slices of bread + 1 cup of milk	1/3 cup of nuts +1 orange + 2 bananas +1 cup of yoghurt	1 cups of cooked brown rice +1 cup cooked vegetables with 10 ml of palm oil + ½ piece of herring
6	3 cups of ready-to-eat oat +1 apple+ 2 bananas +	2 cups of yoghurt	2 cups cooked vegetables with 10 ml of palm oil + a piece of skinless meat
7	2 cups of cooked brown rice +1½ cup of cooked vegetables with 10 ml of palm oil + 1 cup of fruit juice	1 cups of cooked brown rice + ½ cup cooked vegetables + a piece of skinless meat + 1 cup of yoghurt	½ cup of cooked dried beans with 5 ml of palm oil

days below

Below are other precautions to be taken in order to prevent/stop hypertension/high blood pressure:

1. Stop smoking
2. Reduce salt intake to one teaspoon or less per day
3. Stop or reduce intake of alcoholic beverages
4. 15-30 minutes of aerobic physical exercise per day
5. Avoid sedentary lifestyles

CONCLUSION

No one is too young or too old to take care of their heart. Hence, all age groups must adopt measures to prevent the occurence of heart diseases.

Adoption of healthy diet is the most important measure to achieve healthy weight reduction as well as to prevent heart diseases. This means eating meals low in sodium and saturated fats but contain more of fish, nuts, legumes fiber-rich whole grains, skinless poultry, fruits and vegetables.

These are all you need to do to lower your blood pressure. They are very simple practices.

It has been proven that DASH eating plan lowers blood pressure in 14 days.

Also, DASH Diet is not only for controlling blood pressure but it also helps in prevention of stroke, heart disease, kidney stones, cancer and diabetes as it has a high amount of antioxidant rich food.

Thank you for reading this book from the beginning to the end.With 100 percent confidence, I want to assure you that what you have just learnt in this book, especially, in the tables above will guide you towards having a healthy body to lead a good life.

ONLY IF YOU TAKE YOUR TIME TO PUT THEM INTO ACTION.

If you have any question(s) pertaining to this book, your medications, or your health, contact me through:

Email: pharmest@gmail.com

Whatsapp (24 hours): +2348084309551

Call (mon-fri; 5pm-9pm): +2348084309551

Connect with Health Solutions Online

Facebook: www.facebook.com/pharmestcare

Blog: www.pharmest.blogspot.com